The Neurotransmitter Solution Training Manual

John A. Allocca, D.Sc., Ph.D.

Copyright © 2017

THIS BOOK IS FOR DR. ALLOCCA'S STUDENTS ONLY. DO NOT COPY OR DISTRIBUTE.

Updated 3/23/17

Be sure to order the companion DVD to this guidebook.

Published by
Allocca Biotechnology, LLC
Northport, New York
Phone (631) 757-3919
john@allocca.com
www.allocca.com

Printed by Createspace.com

ISBN 978-1544912523

Table of Contents

The Neurotransmitter Solution --3

Low Serotonin and Norepinephrine --4

Effects of Brain Chemistry Imbalance ---5

Brain Chemistry Imbalance ---6

Migraine, Depression, and Other Serotonin and Norepinephrine Disorders -----8

What is the treatment of choice? --9

Migraine Symptoms --10

Brain Chemistry Imbalance --11

Tyramine ---13

Food Allergies --14

Tyramine Containing Food --15

The Neurotransmitter Solution Software --24

Blood Pressure --27

Core Temperature --29

Urinalysis --32

BrainicityTM Transcranial Neural Network Optimizer ---------------------------36

The Neurotransmitter Solution

- Migraine
- Depression
- Insomnia
- Bipolar disorder Excessive aggression Anger and Violence Carbohydrate craving Irritable bowel syndrome Tinnitus
- Fibromyalgia
- Seasonal affective disorder
- More...

Low Serotonin and Norepinephrine

Live a happy and healthy life with Dr. Allocca's Neurotransmitter Protocol!

Diet and Environmental Factors Influence Brain Chemistry, which Influences the Body and Behavior

Effects of Brain Chemistry Imbalance

- Migraine Headaches, Depression, and Insomnia
- Anger, Violence, and Bipolar Syndrome Increased Appetite for Carbohydrates Irritable Bowel Syndrome
- Tinnitus
- Fibromyalgia
- Premenstrual Syndrome
- Seasonal Affective Disorder (SAD) and more

Brain Chemistry Imbalance

Imbalances in your brain chemistry, particularly your neurotransmitter levels, have a large range of effects on your emotions, behavior, brain circulation, and carbohydrate craving.

Neurotransmitters are chemicals that pass signals between nerves. Serotonin and norepinephrine are the two main neurotransmitters used in your brain to control the size of your blood vessels as well as other brain functions.

These neurotransmitter levels in your brain can be diminished by:
- allergic reactions
- inflammation
- poor absorption of nutrients into the brain poor metabolism of nutrients in the brain chemicals that deplete them
- excessive depletion (over usage)
- not enough nutrients to produce more

Migraine, depression, insomnia, bipolar disorder, and carbohydrate craving have similar mechanisms and pathways, all resulting from a loss of brain serotonin and norepinephrine.

If the level of serotonin in the brain is low, one will crave carbohydrates.

Serotonin is manufactured within the brain from the amino acid tryptophan, which is transported into the brain by an albumin carrier.

Proteins and fatty acids compete with tryptophan to get onto this albumin carrier. If one craves and eat carbohydrates, tryptophan will be transported more easily into the brain without much competition from proteins and fatty acids.

The resulting high level of carbohydrates cause other problems.

However, there is another way.

If the brain is supplied with a tryptophan metabolite that transports directly into the brain along with vitamins and minerals needed by the brain to make serotonin, the brain will make serotonin as needed without craving carbohydrates.

The second part of the program is to eliminate foods and substances that cause one to lose serotonin.

We can help increase the level of serotonin and norepinephrine in a natural way.

There are almost always complications, which are addressed using a computer analysis.

Migraine, Depression, and Other Serotonin and Norepinephrine Disorders

Excerpts from the book "What is Your Brain Telling You to Do?"

Cho Seung Hui woke up one morning and was driven out of control to go on a homicidal rampage killing 32 students and faculty members.

Cho Seung Hui was taking antidepressant drugs.

Antidepressants have been used by the perpetrators of similar acts of violence, including the shootings at Columbine High School.

There is a definite relationship between antidepressants and violent acts.

Research on the drug Paxil from the Cardiff University in Britain and the Cochrane Centre in 2006 found that more than twice as many people taking it experienced a serious "hostility event" as did those taking a placebo.

In the United States, labels for all antidepressants note that anxiety, agitation, panic attacks, irritability, hostility, aggressiveness, impulsivity, and mania are all possible side effects.

Furthermore, what was Cho Seung Hui's diet like? Was he eating cheese?

What is the treatment of choice?

The conventional treatment uses drugs (S.S.R.I.s) that force serotonin to remain in the neural junction.

This type of treatment puts the patient at a higher risk of violent behavior.

The alternative treatment is to provide the brain with the nutrients that it needs to make serotonin and norepinephrine, while following a tyramine free diet.

Migraine Symptoms

There are two major classifications of Migraine headaches, with and without visual disturbances.

The Migraine with visual disturbances, which is usually the most severe, is characterized by a visual disturbance, numbness on one side of the body or limb, and/or slight speech abnormality.

These symptoms, referred to as the "aura," will diminish as a headache on the left or right side of the head, nausea, vomiting, etc. become more pronounced.

The visual disturbance may last anywhere from 5 minutes to 30 minutes.

As the visual disturbance slowly disappears, it gives way to boring pain generalized or localized in one area of the head.

The pain will increase in intensity and acquire a throbbing character.

The throbbing characteristic may be intensified by stooping and by all forms of exertion, light, or sound.

If one lies down the intensity may be increased, and it is slightly reduced when sitting upright.

Brain Chemistry Imbalance

Imbalances in brain chemistry, particularly neurotransmitter levels, have a large range of effects on emotions, behavior, and brain circulation.

Brain Chemistry Imbalance

Neurotransmitters are chemical substances that pass signals between nerves.

Serotonin and norepinephrine are the two main neurotransmitters used in the brain to control the size of blood vessels as well as other functions.

These neurotransmitter levels can be diminished by allergic reactions, inflammation, poor absorption of nutrients into the brain, poor metabolism of nutrients in the brain, chemicals that deplete them, excessive depletion (over usage) lowering them or because there are not enough nutrients in the brain to produce more.

Congestive bowel toxicity and intestinal dysbiosis play a major role in producing neurotoxins.

Migraine, depression, and insomnia have similar mechanisms and pathways, all resulting from a loss of serotonin and norepinephrine.

The loss of serotonin and norepinephrine may be quantified in three stages:

Stage 1 is the first level below normal whereby insomnia is experienced.

Stage 2 is the next lower level whereby depression is experienced.

Stage 3 is the next lower level whereby a migraine headache is experienced

Loss of Neurotransmitters

The Neurotransmitter Solution approach to migraine and other serotonin and norepinephrine disorders is twofold:

- Remove the substances that are causing a loss of serotonin and norepinephrine.
- Provide the brain with the raw ingredients it needs to make serotonin and norepinephrine using the NeuroLife formula.

The patented NeuroLife formula has been recommended by physicians during pregnancy.

Tyramine

Tyramine is a vaso-active amino acid that displaces norepinephrine from the nerve endings and epinephrine from the adrenal glands.

Monoamine oxidase, which may be lacking in some individuals, in the gastrointestinal tract inactivates tyramine.

There is an adverse reaction when there is either too much tyramine or too little monoamine oxidase.

The tyramine content in foods vary greatly due to different processing, aging, fermentation, ripening and/or contamination.

Many foods that contain small amounts of tyramine develop large amounts of tyramine if the food products were left to spoil, age (not fresh), or fermented.

The emphasis is placed on FRESH FOODS.

Fruits that are permissible should be very fresh.

Avoid leftovers kept in the refrigerator especially meats, dry packages mixes and can products (prepared foods), yeast extracts, and protein extracts.

Remember, foods increase in their tyramine content as they age or ferment.

For example, bananas are permissible if they are fresh, not if they are overripe.

Tyramine can also be produced by bacteria in the gastrointestinal track.

Helicobactor pylori can produce large amounts of tyramine in the gut.

Various bacteria, such as high dose probiotics, in the gut can cause an increase in the production of tyramine.

Food Allergies

Eating any food one is allergic to can cause migraine headaches and other neurotransmitter problems.

If in doubt, see an allergist for food allergy testing.

Food allergies may include, but not limited to the following:
- Eggs, If allergic
- Wheat, if allergic
- Corn, if allergic
- Milk, if allergic
- Soy, if allergic
- Anything else, if allergic

Tyramine Containing Food

Food is fermented using bacteria, which produce tyramine, a chemical that causes migraine headaches and other problems.

This includes the following:

Primary (absolutely avoid):

- Any Food that is Aged, Cultured, Fermented, or naturally contains Tyramine
- Cheeses Chocolate
- Yogurt Over-ripened fruits

Secondary (small amounts may be tolerated):

- Citrus and Citric Acid
- Berries (most kinds with thick skin) Red Plums
- Pineapple
- Raisins
- Raspberries
- Bananas
- Grapes
- Apples
- Figs
- Tomatoes
- Raw Onions
- Avocado
- Spinach
- Green Pepper
- Chili Peppers
- Nuts and nut butters Coconut and coconut-oil

- Many Beans and Peas
- Frankfurters, bacon, etc. containing nitrates Sourdough
- Carob
- Most teas are fermented
- Garlic
- Wine
- Cold cuts containing nitrates, etc.
- Salad bars that spray with sulfites
- Aged, marinated, or pickled meats Smoked/cured meats
- Non-fresh meats or fish
- Tofu
- Smoked fish
- Mustard
- Red wine
- Alcoholic beverages including beer Caffeine greater than 300 mg per day
- Tempeh
- Tomari
- Umbusi
- Soy sauce Miso
- Vinegar Tobacco Protein extracts Ginseng Ginger

Chemicals that cause loss of neurotransmitters:
- Monosodium Glutamate (MSG)
- Nitrates & Nitrites
- Meat tenderizers
- Aspartame (nutrasweet)
- Saccharin (includes toothpaste and mouthwash) Food preservatives

- Yeast and brewers extracts Frequent use of amphetamines
- Frequent use of barbituates Frequent use of recreation drugs
- Decaffeinated coffee (only 50% less caffeine)
- Paint fumes & other chemical fumes
- Some drugs can trigger a migraine, Depression, etc. depending upon your sensitivity to those drugs
- Excessive exposure to fluorescent lighting

Food to Eat:

- The following food are relatively safe to eat unless your are allergic to any of them.
- YOUR DIET IS NOT LIMITED TO THOSE ITEMS BELOW
- Bell & Evans Frozen Fully Cooked Grilled Chicken Breasts, Frozen, Ingredients: boneless, skinless,chicken beasts, water, sea salt, rice starch.
- Lundberg Organic brown rice, short or long grain, Ingredients: organic short or long grain brown rice.
- Lundberg Organic brown basmati rice, Ingredients: organic California brown basmati rice.
- Minute Ready to Serve brown rice, Ingredients: water, whole grain brown rice, soybean oil, salt, soy lecithin.
- Shiloh Farms Organic Potato Fakes, instant, Ingredients: organic potato flakes, monoglycerides, and diglycerides (from organic palm oil).
- Any brand, Instant Oatmeal or regular oatmeal, Ingredients: whole grain instant oats.
- Nature's Path Organic Crispy Rice, Ingredients: brown rice flour, evaporated cane juice, sea salt, molasses.
- Quaker Rice Cakes, Ingredients: whole grain brown rice.
- Romain Lettuce, broccoli, zucchini, carrots, and many other vegetables, except raw garlic, onions, and radishes.
- Cold Pressed Olive Oil.

- Coffee, unflavored, organic. Organic Fat-Free Milk if not allergic.
- Organic Butter in small quantities. Ice Cream, vanilla.
- Spices: parsley, oregano, basil, pepper, salt, in small quantity.
- Sweetener: sugar in small quantity.

Serotonin Pathways

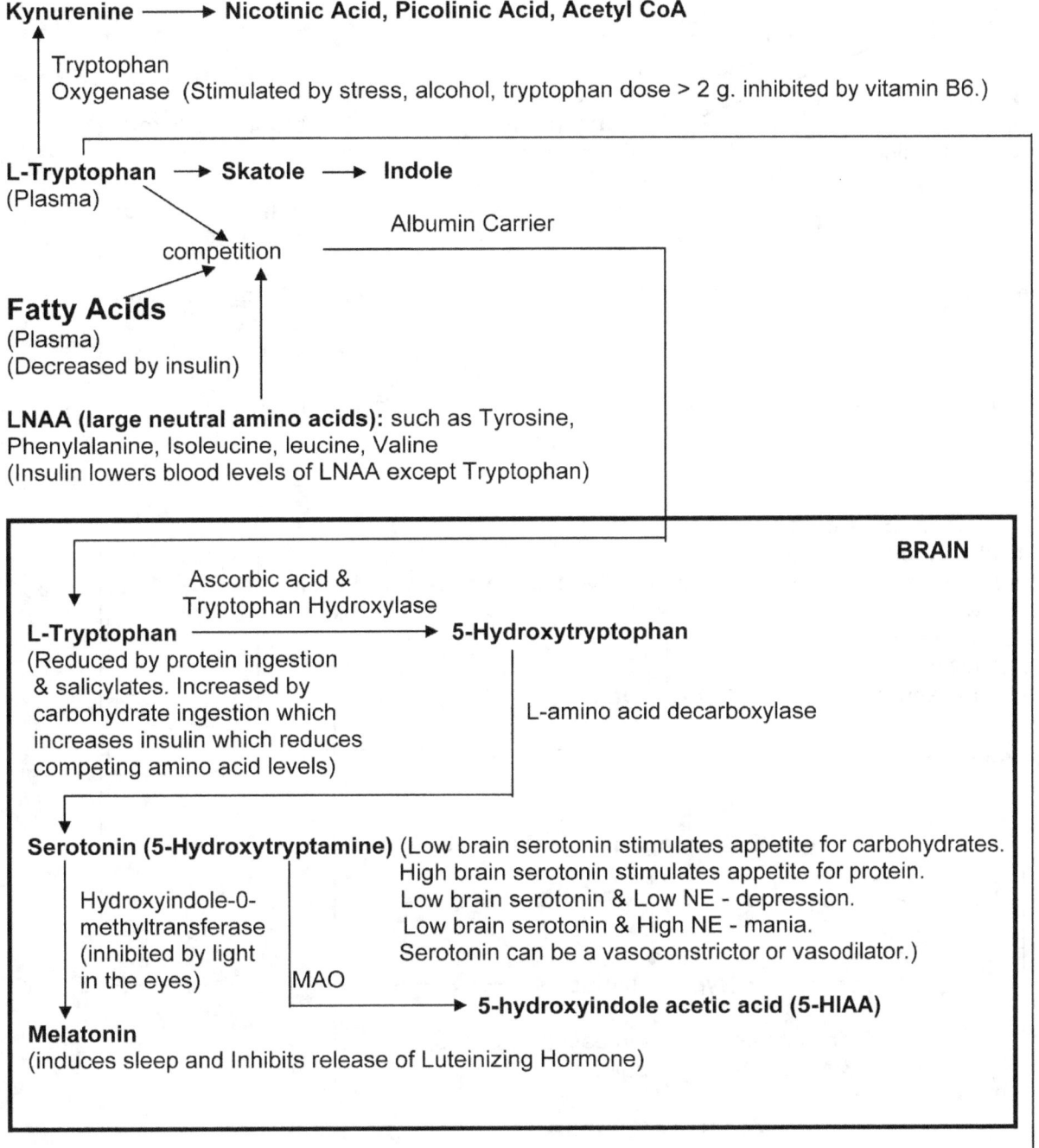

Continued on next page

Migraine Pathways

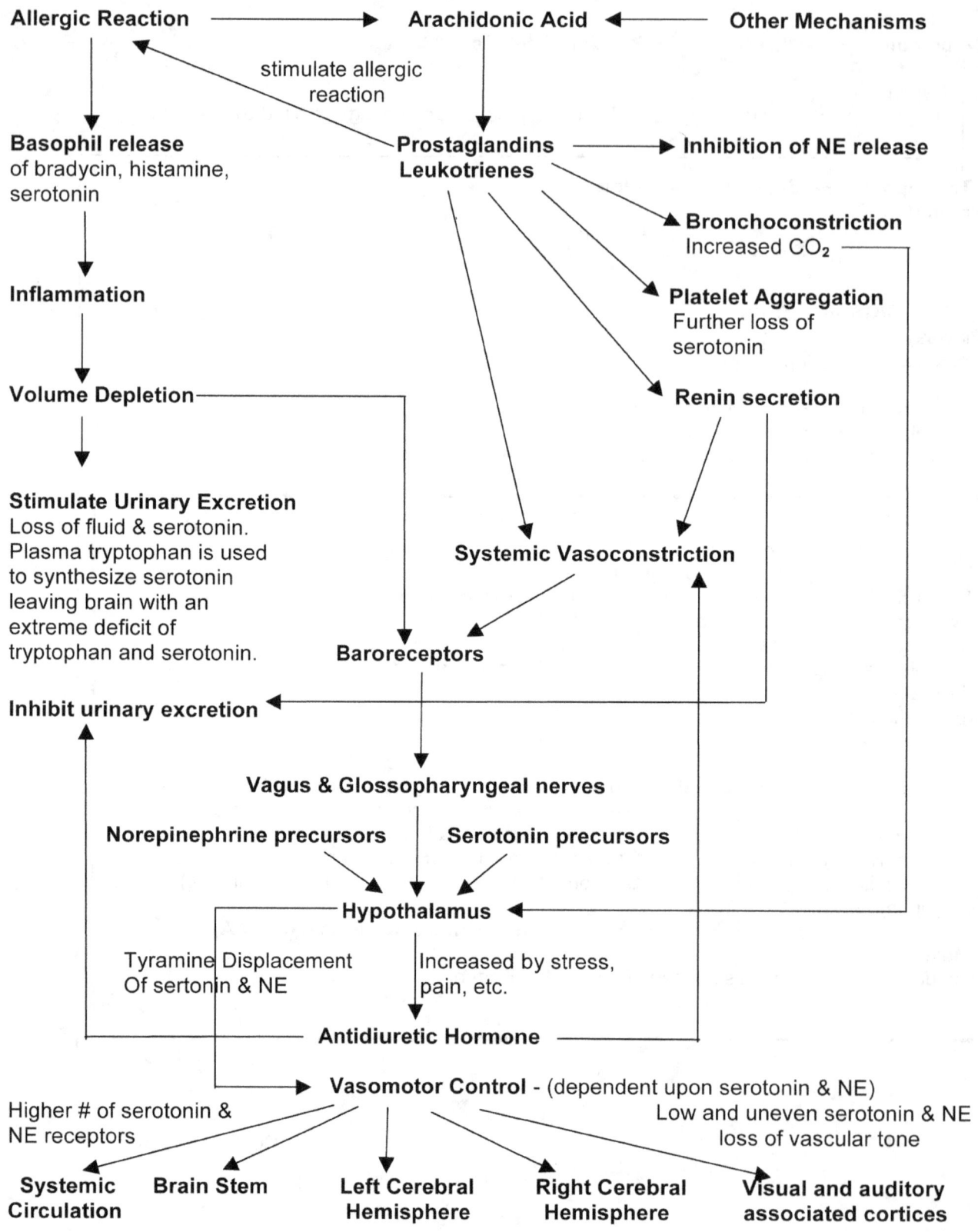

Depression Pathways

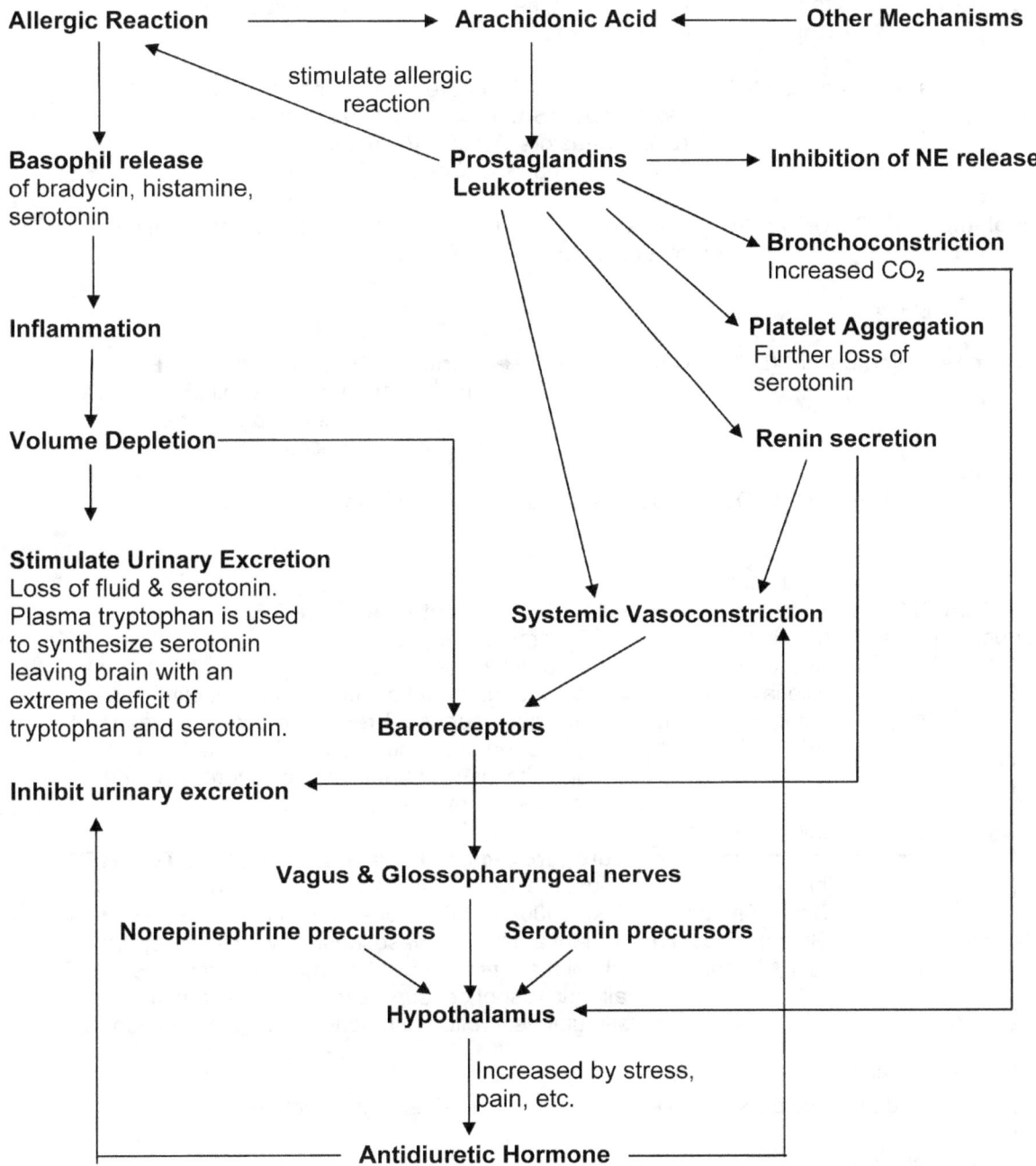

21

Omega 6 Fatty Acid - Eicosanoid Pathways

Linoleic Acid (LA) C18:2w6 (sunflower, safflower, corn, sesame, seed and vegetable oils, legumes, mother's milk, etc.)

    ↓   Delta-6-Desaturase (D6D) (D6D is inhibited by adrenaline, Alpha-Linolenic Acid, and blocked by NSAID's, Steroids, & alcohol)
(D6D co-factors include: Vitamins A, B6, C, Folic acid, and Zinc, Copper, Magnesium)

Gamma-Linolenic acid (GLA) C18:3w6 (borage oil, evening primrose oil, black current oil, pumpkin, mother's milk)

    ↓   Elongase

Dihomo-Gamma-Linolenic Acid (DGLA) C20:3w6 ⟶ **Series 1: Prostaglandin (PGE1)**, (anti-inflammatory, vasodilative, blocks allergic response, improves nerve function, enhances immune function)

    ↓   Delta-5-Desaturase (D5D) (D5D is stimulated by Insulin, and inhibited by glucagon & EPA)

Arachidonic Acid C20:4w6 (animal products)

    Cyclooxygenase ⟶ **Series 2: Prostaglandin (PGE2)**, Thromboxane (A2),
(blocked by NSAID's, Bioflavonoids, Ginger, Vitamin E EPA, Zinc)
(pro-inflammatory, vasoconstrictive, tissue repair, platelet aggregation, clot formation, stimulates allergic response & renin secretion, increases glycogenolysis, suppresses immune function, inhibits insulin release, inhibits norepinephrine release from synaptic junction)

    Lipoxygenase ⟶ **Hydroperoxyeicosatetraenoic acid, (HPETE), (HETE),** Leukotrienes (LT) - 1000x more powerful than PGE's, A's, 1,000-10,000x more inflammatory than histamine
(blocked by Bioflavonoids, Ginger, Vitamin E, Zinc, Selenium, EPA)
(pro-inflammatory, vasoconstrictive, tissue repair, platelet aggregation, clot formation, stimulates allergic response, suppresses immune function, stimulate secretion of mucus, airway constriction.)

Phospholipase (blocked by Steroids & Vitamin E, stimulated by IgE allergic reactions)

Membrane Phospholipids

Nerve Stimulus ⟶ Norepinephrine release ⟶ PGE2
(inhibited by PGE2 at pre-synaptic junction) ⟵

Figure 10 – Balancing Serotonin and Norepinephrine

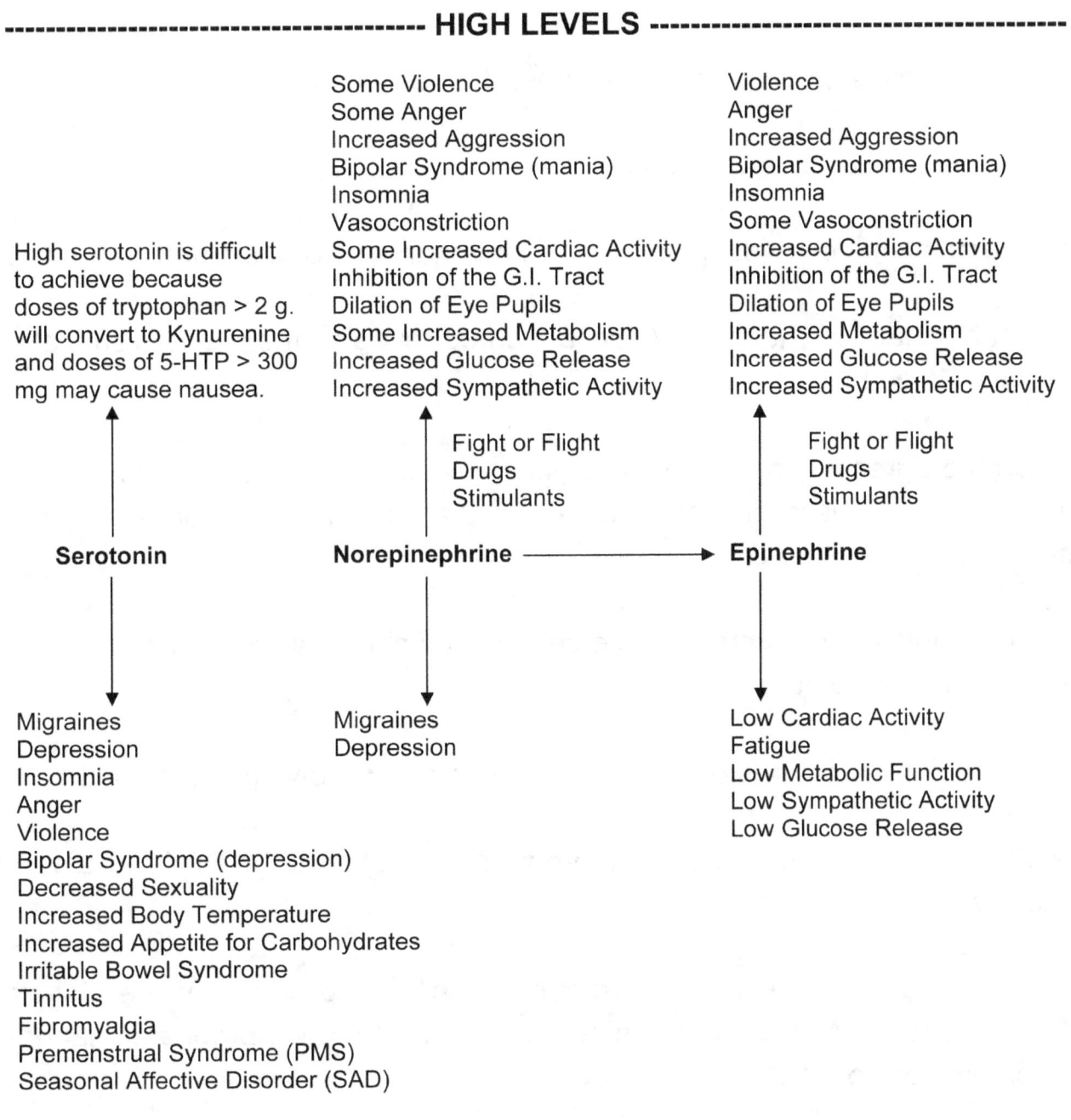

Notes: The effects of epinephrine last 5-10 times longer and have a greater effect on metabolism and cardiac stimulation than norepinephrine, and have a weaker effect on vasoconstriction / increased blood pressure. The dynamics of neurotransmitter levels must be analyzed with respect to time. Changes in neurotransmitter levels begins with an initial reaction followed by a loss of neurotransmitter reserves if they cannot be replaced at least at the rate by which they are depleted.

The Neurotransmitter Solution Software

It all started with a solution to migraine headaches.

Then, more solutions were created.

A biochemical model reveals the complex mechanisms of a biological process.

The first biochemical model Dr. Allocca created revealed the mechanisms of migraine headaches.

Research progressed to developing biochemical models for depression, insomnia, bipolar disorder, violence, carbohydrate craving, membrane transport systems, and much more.

Then, Dr. Allocca programmed these complex biochemical models into a state-of-the-art software program.

The software program has evolved and is constantly evolving since 1996.

The biochemical models used in the program are published in Dr. Allocca's textbooks.

The Neurotransmitter Solution program produces an individualized step-by-step plan geared towards each person's needs to facilitate the appropriate changes for problems discovered.

The Neurotransmitter Solution data processing service is available to healthcare professionals.

Conditions Addressed:

- Migraine Prevention Depression
- Insomnia
- Bipolar disorder
- Excessive Aggression
- Anger and Violence Carbohydrate Craving Decreased Sexuality Increased Body Temperature Irritable Bowel Syndrome
- Tinnitus
- Fibromyalgia
- Premenstrual Syndrome
- Seasonal Affective Disorder
- Weight Problems
- Poor Digestion and Malabsorption Hormonal Imbalances
- Irritable Bowel Syndrome
- Intestinal Candida (yeast) Overgrowth Allergies
- Pre and Post Menopausal Syndrome Nutritional Deficiencies
- Inflammation
- Arthritis
- Adrenal Imbalances
- Thyroid Imbalances
- Diabetes
- and much more...

Tests/Information
- Age
- Sex
- Height and Weight
- Blood Pressure
- Daytime Core Temperature Urinalysis
- Symptoms Questionnaire

Report
- Client Information
- Conditions which may Interfere with Good Health Calculated Basal Metabolic Rate
- Calculated Body Mass Index
- Daytime Core Temperature
- Symptoms Probability Profile (color bar graph) Urinalysis with Explanations
- Systems Evaluation
- Recommendations (food, exercise, & supplements)

Data Processing Service

The Data Processing Service is just so easy. Simply fax or mail us the completed data form.

We will process the data and send you a complete analysis and plan in pdf format via email.

Forms can be downloaded from www.allocca.com

Blood Pressure

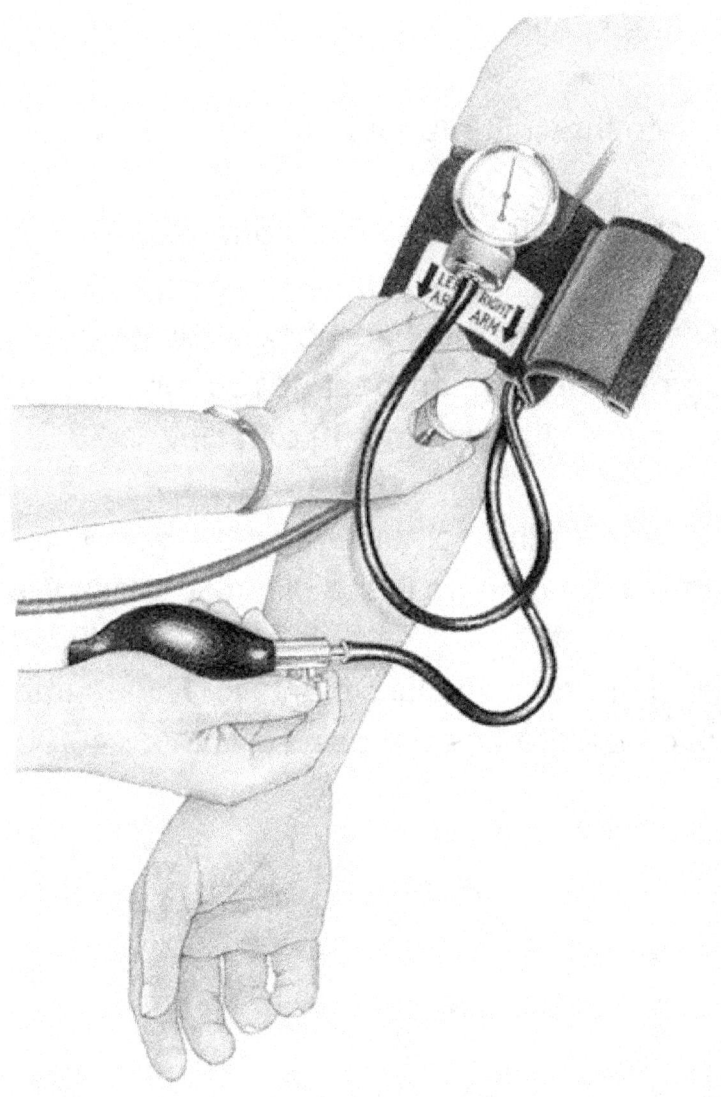

1. A sphygmomanometer (blood pressure cuff, valve, and gage) of the appropriate size and stethoscope will be required.

2. Apply the cuff around the patients arm approximately one inch above the elbow. Be sure to place the artery arrow inline with the brachial artery.

3. Place the stethoscope on the brachial artery at the anterior joint of the elbow. This is the point where the artery is closest to the surface. Place the other end of the stethoscope in your ears. Note that your ear canal is not straight into your

head, but rather at angle towards the front. Your stethoscope should be inserted at this angle.

4. Tighten the valve on the sphygmomanometer.

5. Pump the bulb to inflate the cuff to about 150 mm Hg, while watching the dial.

6. Gently release the valve slightly to let the air out slowly.

7. Watch the dial and listen for the first heart beat. This is the systolic pressure. Remember it. If you do not hear a heart beat at 150 mm Hg, repeat the procedure and pump the cuff higher than 150 mm Hg.

8. Listen as the air releases for the point at which the sound disappears. The point just before the sound disappears is the diastolic pressure. Remember it.

9. Write down the two numbers as systolic/diastolic. For example, 120/70. High blood pressure is considered as a pressure above 140/90.

Core Temperature

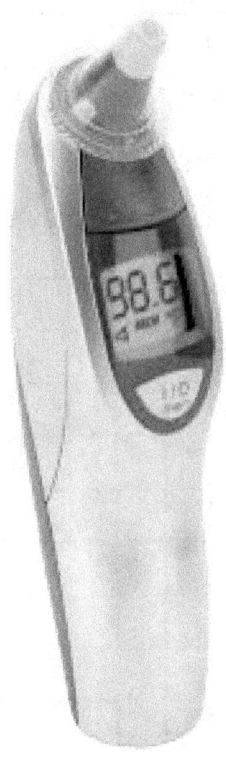

Normal Body Temperature

Previously, average oral temperature for healthy adults had been considered 98.6 degrees F, while the normal ranges is 97.0 to 100.0 degrees F.

Recent studies suggest that the average temperature for healthy adults is 98.2 degrees F.

Daily activity plays an important role in body temperature.

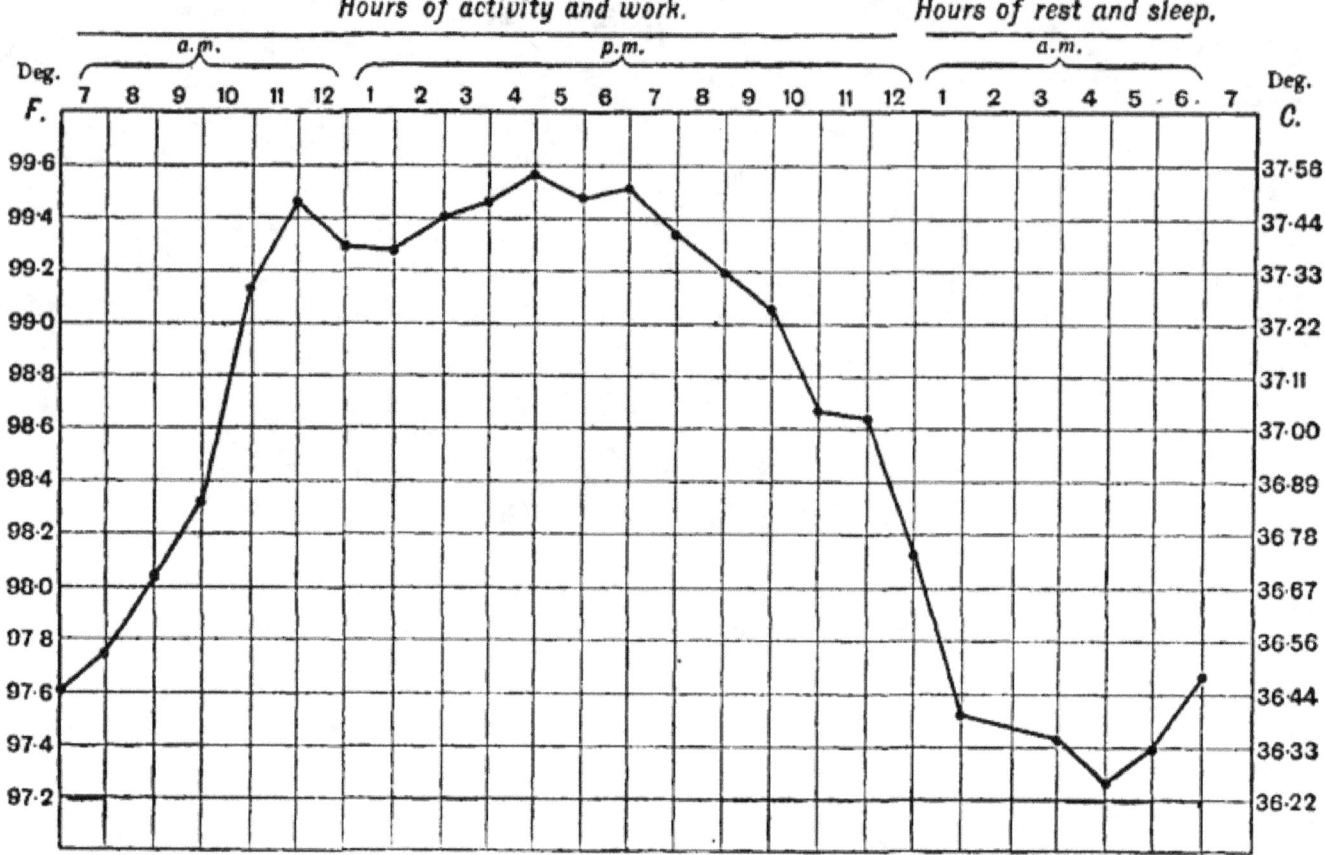

From 7 am to 1 am (chart above):

Normal Daytime Core Temperature (Ear): 97.8 to 99.6 F (36.6-37.6 C)

Within 24 hours of ovulation, women experience an elevation of 0.2 - 0.9 F due to the increased metabolic rate caused by sharply elevated levels of progesterone.

Women can chart this phenomenon to determine whether and when they are ovulating, so as to aid conception or contraception.

During strenuous exercise or extreme emotions, excessive body heat is produced.

Body Temperature can temporarily rise as high as 101 to 104 F.
When the body is exposed to extreme cold, the body temperature can fall to below 96 F.

The Braun ThermoScan Pro 4000 electronic ear thermometer is the instrument of choice for reliable measuring of core temperature.

Studies have show the ear thermometer to be a reliable source for measuring core temperature.

Basal Temperature Test for Thyroid Function

Basal (resting) body temperature is based on the work of Broda O. Barnes, M.D. during the 1970's
Dr. Barnes correlated basal body temperature with basal metabolism on thousands of patients.

A basal temperature below 97.8 F (36.6 C) strongly suggests under-active thyroid function.

A basal temperature above 98.2 F (36.8 C) strongly suggests an infection or overactive thyroid function.

Urinalysis

A Fresh sample should be used.

No food 4 hours before test.

No alcohol 24 hours before test.

Appearance

Normal urine is clear.

Cloudy urine indicates infectious solutes (WBC's, pus, bacteria) or it is too alkaline.

Color

Colorless indicates a high water intake or anemia or bile deficiency. Yellow is normal.

Dark Yellow indicates dehydration or antibiotic use or Vitamins A, B supplements or fasting and has high fever.

Yellow-brown or Yellow-green indicates bile pigments in urine or from drugs.

Red or Red-brown caused by eating beets or hemoglobin in the urine or from some medications.

Orange-red or Orange-brown indicates presence of urobilinogen in the urine or from drugs.

Dark-brown or Black indicates malanins or dark pigments of tumors in the urinary tract or the presence of iron portion of hemoglobin in the urine.

Specific Gravity (1.016 - 1.022)

Osmolality (concentration). Above 1.022 indicates renal dysfunction or dehydration.

pH (5 - 7)

Above 7 indicates metabolic alkalosis or infection or diet high in alkaline ash. Below 5 indicates metabolic acidosis or high stress or excessive stimulants (Caffeine, alcohol, drugs).

Leukocytes (0)

Positive indicates infection or high Vitamin C intake.
Nitrite (0)

Bacteria convert nitrate to nitrite in the urine. Presence of nitrite indicates bacterial infection of the kidney or urinary tract.

Protein (0 - 30 mg/dl)

Above 30 mg/dl indicates renal dysfunction or excessive protein in the diet or strenuous exercise or emotional stress or during fever or exposure to excessive heat or cold. Protein in the urine for a prolonged period of time indicates renal dysfunction.

Glucose (0)

The kidney's will reabsorb all the glucose in the urine as long as the level is below 160 - 190 mg%. Positive glucose in the urine indicates diabetes.

Ketones (0)

When glucose is not available during fasting, adipose tissue triglycerides are reconverted to free fatty acids and glycerol (lipolysis). When the fatty acids are metabolized, ketone bodies are produced as an energy source for the brain and other tissues when glucose is not available. Positive indicates fasting or carbohydrate starvation or vomiting or diarrhea or diabetes or excessive alcohol use.

Urobilinogen (less than 1 mg/dl)

Increased blood cell destruction increases bilirubin and the subsequent conversion to urobilinogen.

Above 1 indicates hemolytic anemia or pernicious anemia or sickle cell anemia Bacteria in the intestinal tract reduce bilirubin to urobilinogen. Urobilinogen is present in the urine in trace amounts. Antibiotics and drugs destroy the intestinal flora and cause an absence of urobilinogen in the urine and feces. It is also absent in obstructive jaundice where no bilirubin reaches the intestinal tract to be converted to urobilinogen.

Absence indicates reduced intestinal flora or liver dysfunction or biliary obstruction.

Bilirubin (0 - 0.5 mg/dl)

Positive indicates liver dysfunction or biliary obstruction.

Bilirubin is formed as result of the breakdown of damaged or worn out red blood cells in the spleen and bone marrow. After hemoglobin is released, it is converted into globin and heme. Heme is converted to bilirubin after the iron is removed for recycling. After passing through the liver, the protein-bound bilirubin is made water soluble and passes into the intestines through the bile duct where it emulsifies fats. When found in the urine, it indicates excess bilirubin in the blood.

Blood (0 - 5 Erythrocytes/ul)

There should not be any red blood cells (erythrocytes) in the urine.
Positive indicates menstruation or infection or strenuous exercise or exposure to excessive cold or renal dysfunction or drugs. Follow up with microscopic exam.

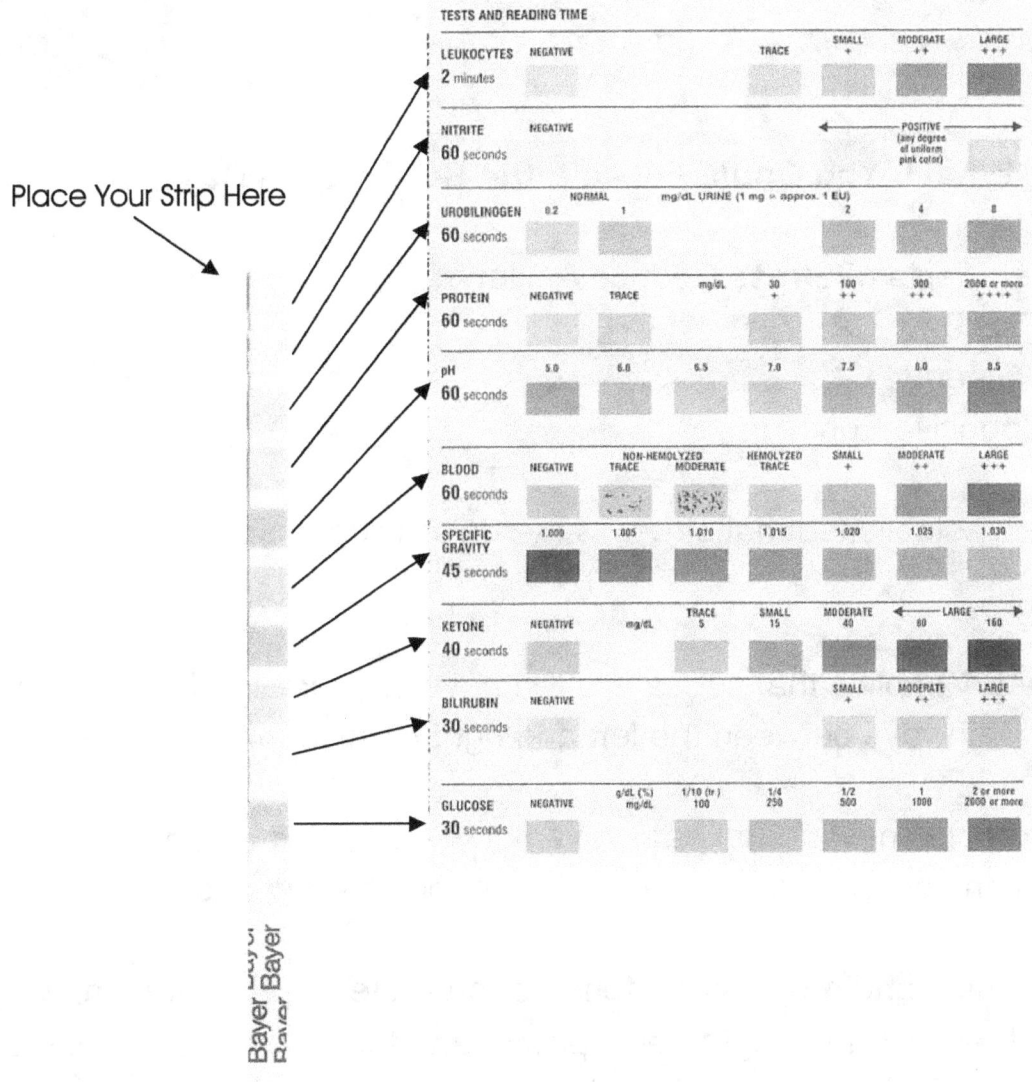

Bayer Multistix 10 SG Reagent Strip Urinalysis
Manufacturer's Number 2161

Brainicity™ Transcranial Neural Network Optimizer

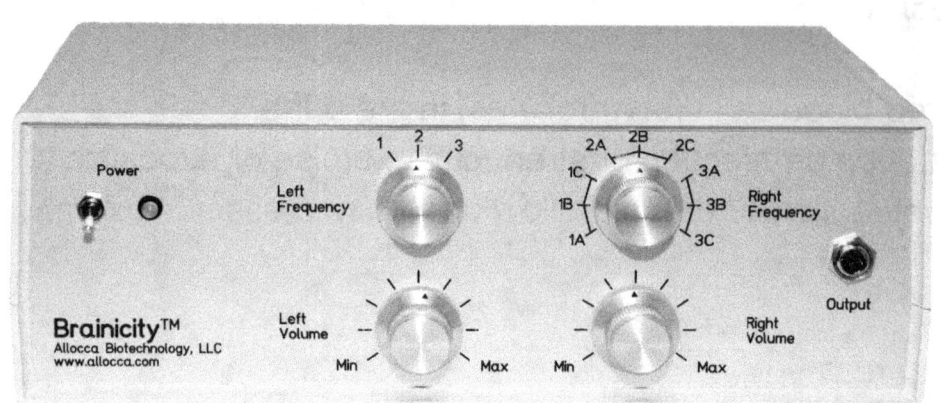 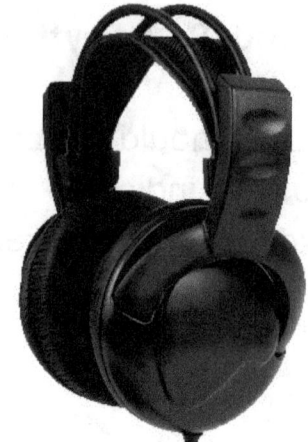

What if You Could Feel a Little Better Each Day?

- Reduce the Effects of Stress Reduce Anxiety
- Reduce P.T.S.D
- Get Better Sleep
- Increase Cognitive Function

It has long been established that stress is the underlying cause of many diseases.

The Allocca theory implies that stress is often not well processed if the brain is lacking neural pathways between the left and right hemispheres

Brainicity™ promotes new neural pathways between the left and right hemispheres of the brain to facilitate the efficient processing of stress.

Brainicity™ is a safe and drugless system that promotes new neural pathways between the left hemisphere, right hemisphere, and the limbic system of the brain for improved Brain Function, Creativity, and Stress Reduction.

Brainicity™ Transcranial Neural Network Optimizer

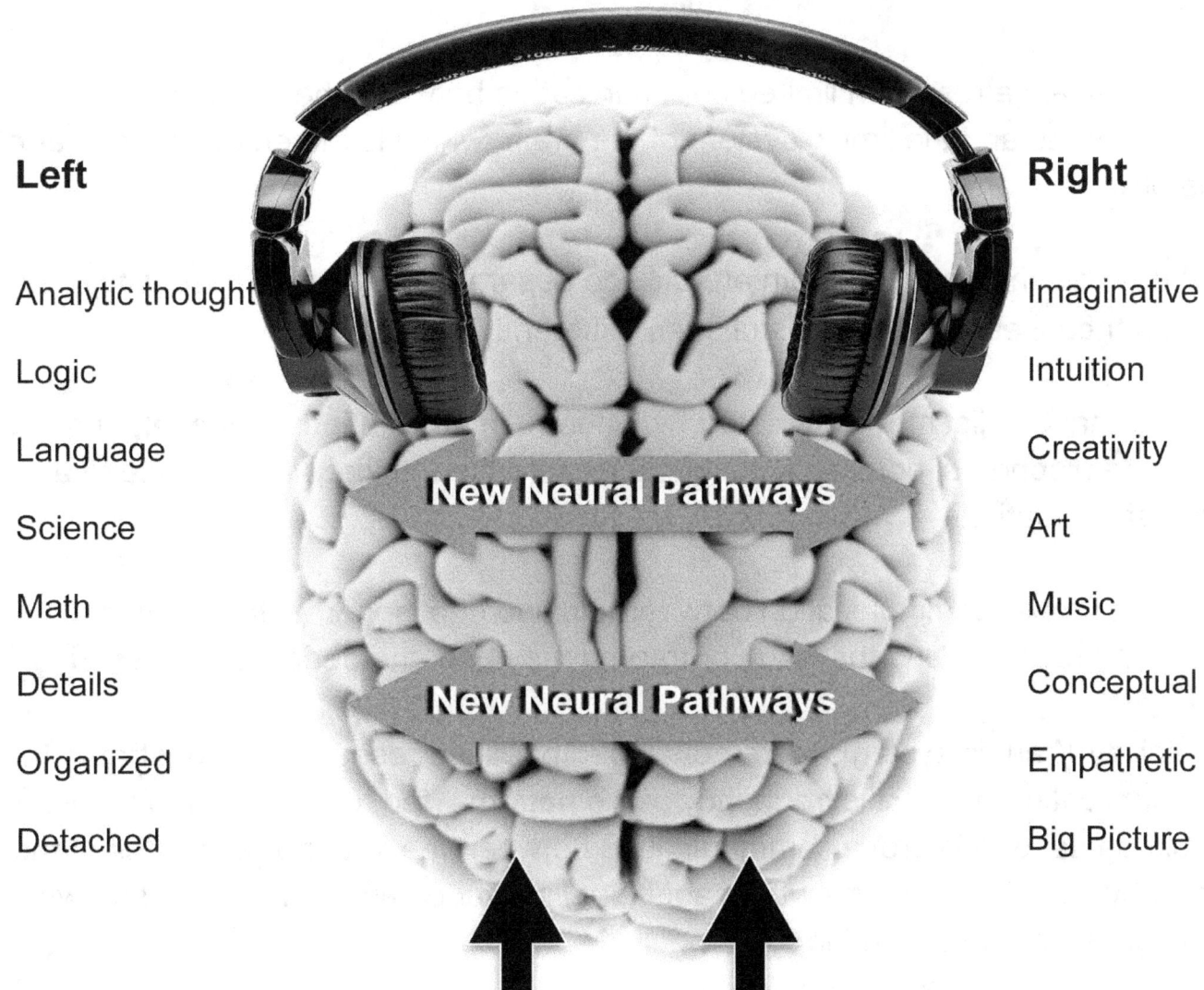

The theory is simple.

The cerebral cortex of the brain is divided into two parts, the left hemisphere and right hemisphere.

Then, those hemispheres interact individually with the limbic system.

The left hemisphere of the brain is primarily used, while the right hemisphere, which is believed to be the center of creative thought, is not used to its fullest capacity.

This imbalance results in limited communication between the left and right hemispheres and the limbic system of the brain, which is the emotional center of the brain.

If the hemispheres of the brain are utilized separately, they may cope with experiences, especially stressful ones, differently.

An internal conflict may be created by different interpretations of the left and right brain hemispheres, potentially resulting in increased anxiety in response to a stressful situation.

Without proper communication between the two hemispheres, the conflict may never be resolved and the issue or trauma may become deeply suppressed.

Brainicity™ audio systems were developed because research demonstrated that the application of specific frequency audio patterns, fed through headphones, could be used to improve communication between the left and right sides of the brain by stimulating the growth of additional neural pathways between the two hemispheres and the limbic system.

In binaural stimulation, two different audio patterns are fed simultaneously through headphones to the left and right ears.
The brain will produce a third pattern that is the difference between the two.

It is this process of binaural stimulation that leads to the production of new neural pathways between the right and left hemispheres of the brain and the limbic system.

Brainicity™ CDs were made from the the BrainicityTM device.

Three common base frequencies that our test subjects chose was used to make the CDs.

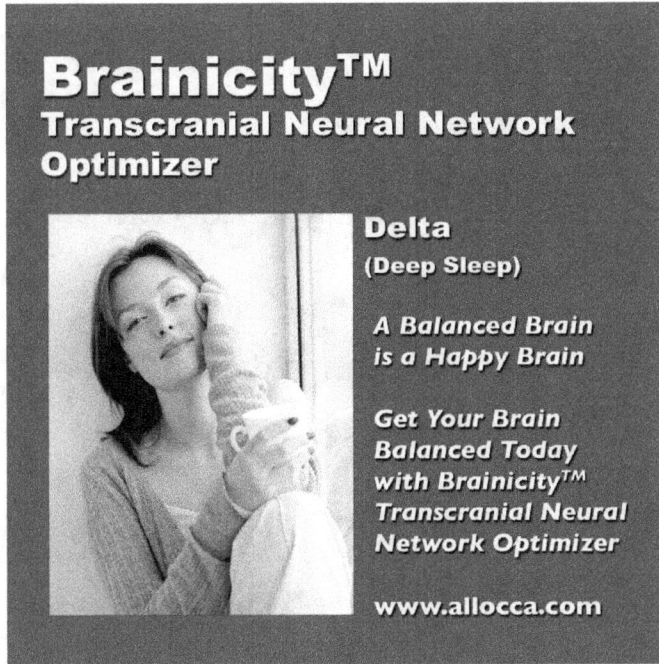
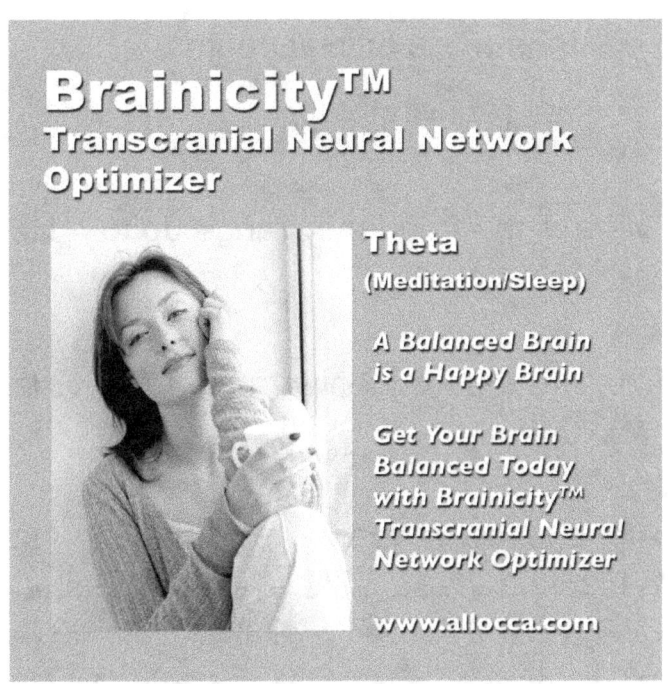
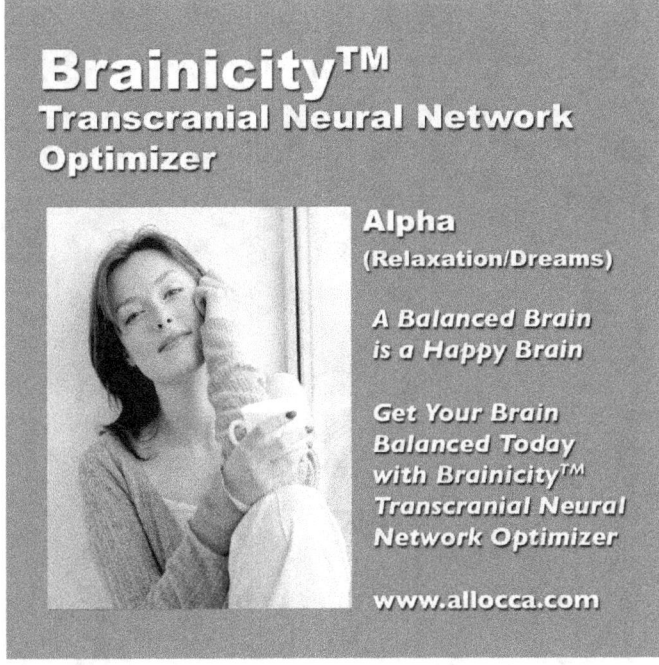
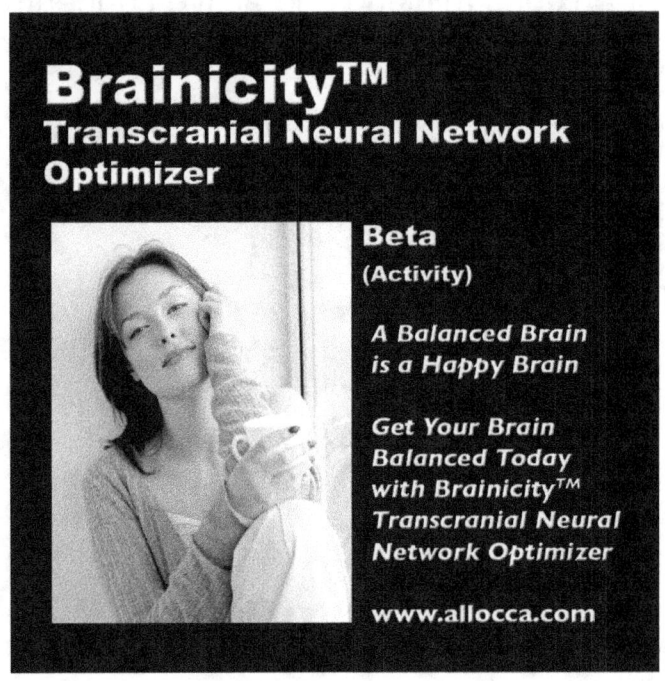

Each CD contains all three base frequencies.

There are four CDs in the series: Delta, Theta, Alpha and Beta.

- Delta (Deep Sleep)
- Theta (Meditation/Sleep)
- Alpha (Relaxation/Dreams)
- Beta (Activity)

Delta is the frequency range up to 4 Hz., which is seen normally in slow wave sleep.

Theta is the frequency range from 4 Hz to 7 Hz., which is seen in drowsiness or meditation.

Alpha is the frequency range from 7 Hz to 14 Hz., which is seen in deep relaxation, closing the eyes, or meditation.

Beta is the frequency range from 15 Hz to 30 Hz., which is seen in active, busy or anxious thinking and active concentration.

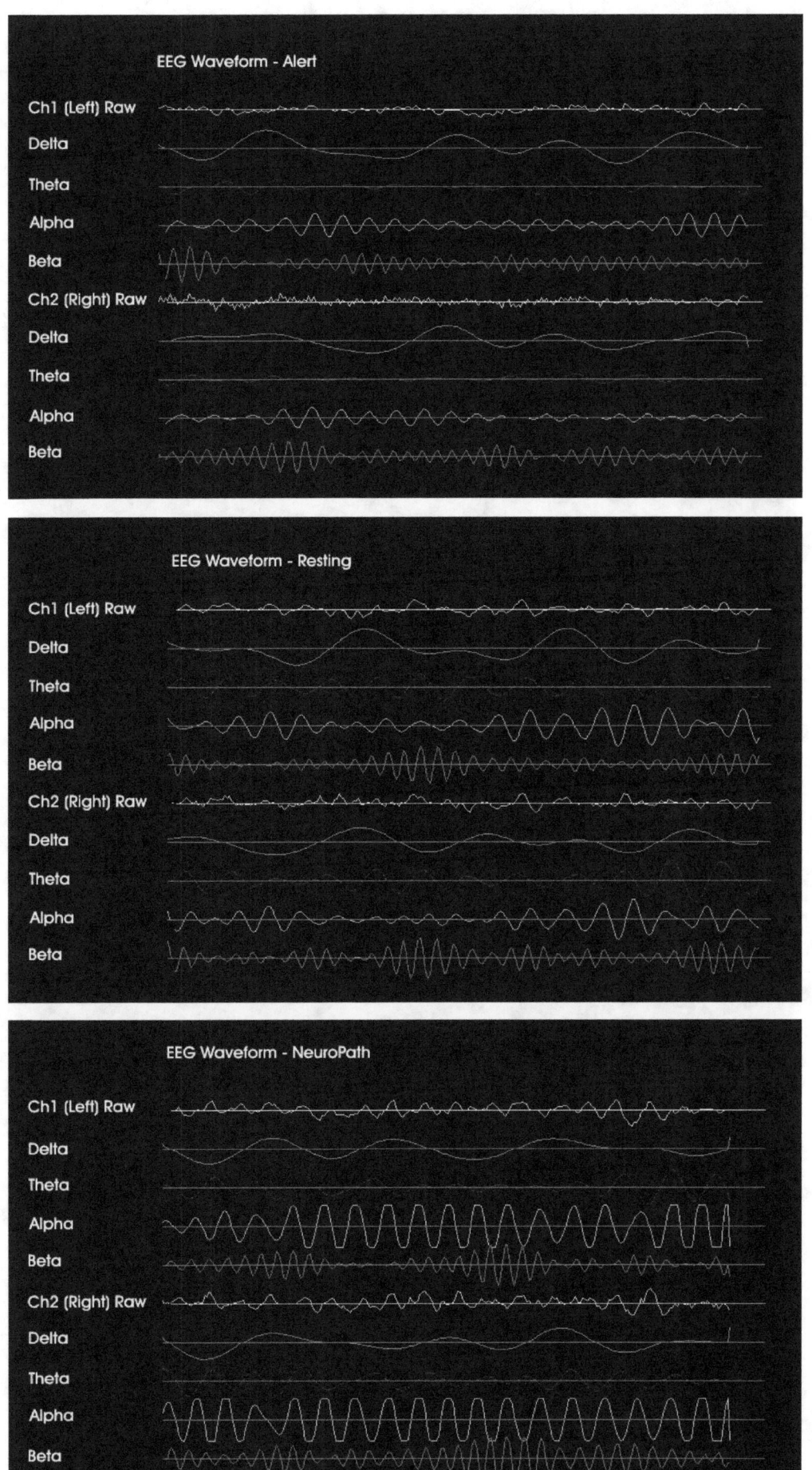

For more information...
John A. Allocca, D.Sc., Ph.D. Medical Research Scientist
Allocca Biotechnology, LLC Northport, NY
(631) 757-3919
www.allocca.com

www.ingramcontent.com/pod-product-compliance
Lightning Source LLC
Chambersburg PA
CBHW081310180526
45170CB00007B/2647